EMBRACE
the Wave

Three Steps to Managing Distressed Emotions and Anxiety

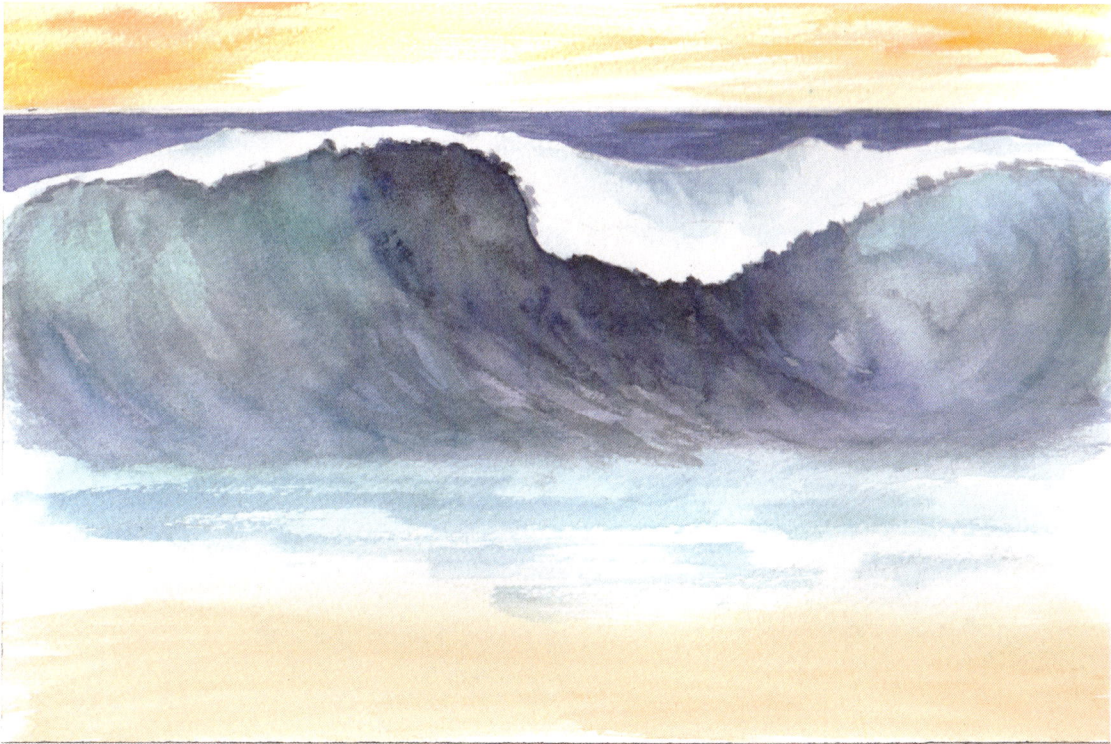

Robin Ingram

Illustrated by Jennifer Hunt

ABOUT THE AUTHOR

Robin S. Ingram, EdM is the Owner and CEO of a local New Mexico based counseling agency. Her credentials include Licensed Professional Clinical Counselor (LPCC), Licensed School Counselor (Level 3) K-12, and Licensed School Administrator K-12.

Ms. Ingram has a proven record of success as a Licensed Family Counselor, Therapist and Educator with ages 3-103. Her expertise includes Children and Adult Individual and Group Counseling, Social/Emotional Support, Programs Development, Community Collaboration and Outreach, Classroom Presentations, Parent Classes and Professional Workshops.

The areas of specialties include; Behavioral Regulation, ADD, ADHD, OCD, ODD, Anxiety, Depression, Trauma, Eating Disorders, Harm to Self-Behaviors, Grief and Loss, Gifted Challenges, Emotional Dysregulation, Pet Grief Support, Insomnia, Diet and Nutrition, Chronic Pain, Depression, Couples Counseling, Parenting Supports, Social Anxiety, Language Development, Academic Supports, Bi Polar, Education and Career Planning.

Therepeutic Interventions Include; Play Therapy, Equine Therapy, Animal Therapy, Art Therapy, Cognitive Reframing, Communication Skills, Compliance Issues, DBT (Dialetic Behavior Therapy) and CBT (Cognative Behavior Therapy), MST (Multi Systems Therapy), Exploration of Coping Patterns, Exploration of Emotions, Exploration of Relationship Patterns, Mindfulness Training, Preventative Services, Psycho-Education, Role-Play/ Behavioral Rehearsal, Interactive Feedback, Preventative Services, Structured Problem Solving, Supportive Reflection and Symptom Management.

Ms. Ingram's Out Reach Supports Include: Workshops, On-site Presentations, On-site visits to Nursing homes, Hospitals and Medical Clinics, Collaboration Meetings, Trainings, Video Classes and Workshops, In-home Visits, and Concierge Options.

Ms. Ingram is delighted to create this much-needed quick-start guide and share her knowledge with all those who seek help.

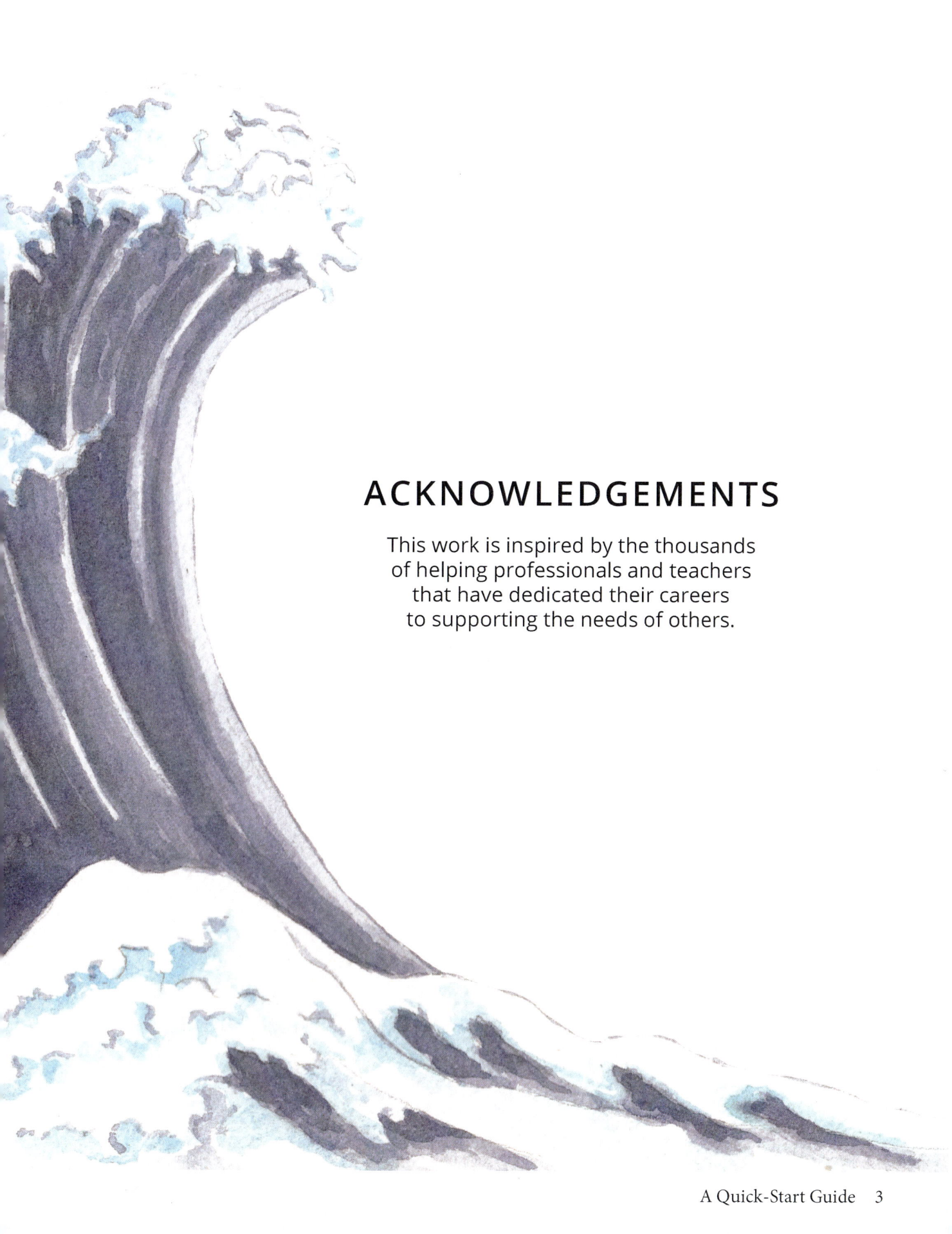

ACKNOWLEDGEMENTS

This work is inspired by the thousands
of helping professionals and teachers
that have dedicated their careers
to supporting the needs of others.

EMBRACE THE WAVE

THE BEGINNINGS…

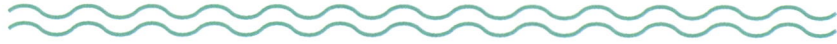

The Waves of the Ocean are like the Waves of Emotion…
They come and go naturally and with different levels of intensity….

Much like we can't prevent the waves reaching the shore, we can't stop our emotions from reaching our minds. Instead of trying to prevent these waves of emotion from reaching us, we need to Embrace them by managing these in a healthy sustainable way.

This book provides you with a systematic approach to acknowledging and respecting your emotions as they affect you throughout the days, weeks and years of your life!

Learn How To Embrace The Waves of YOUR Emotions!
Let's Get Started NOW!

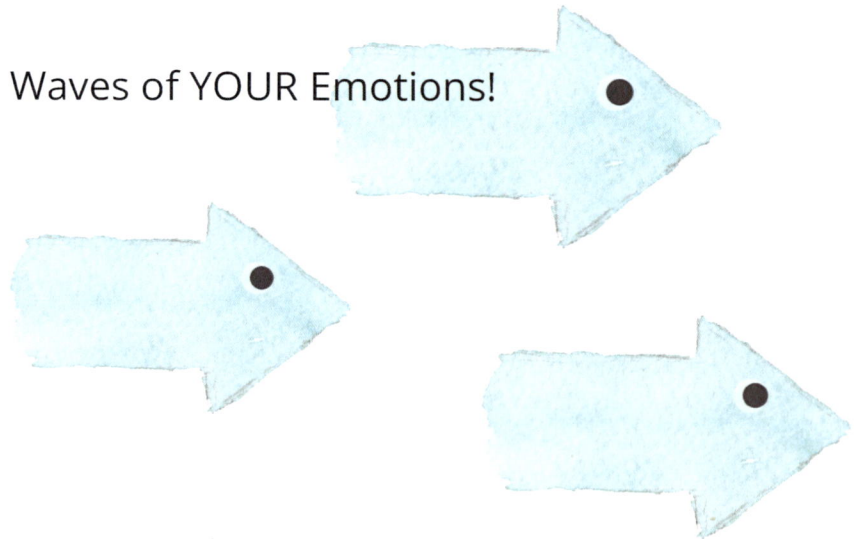

Step 1:

IDENTIFYING FEELINGS AND TRIGGER

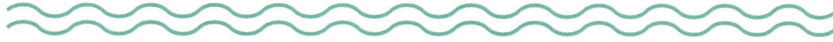

~~~~~~~~~~~~~~~~~~~~

• Acknowledge your emotions by describing them in detail: I am feeling ...

  Frustrated, Enraged, Nervous, Irritated, Terrified, Confused, Sad, Anxious, Impatient, Annoyed, Angry, Self Conscious etc.

• Stand up and walk to another space with your Journal.

• Write down your emotions and what triggered this in step one of your Journal.

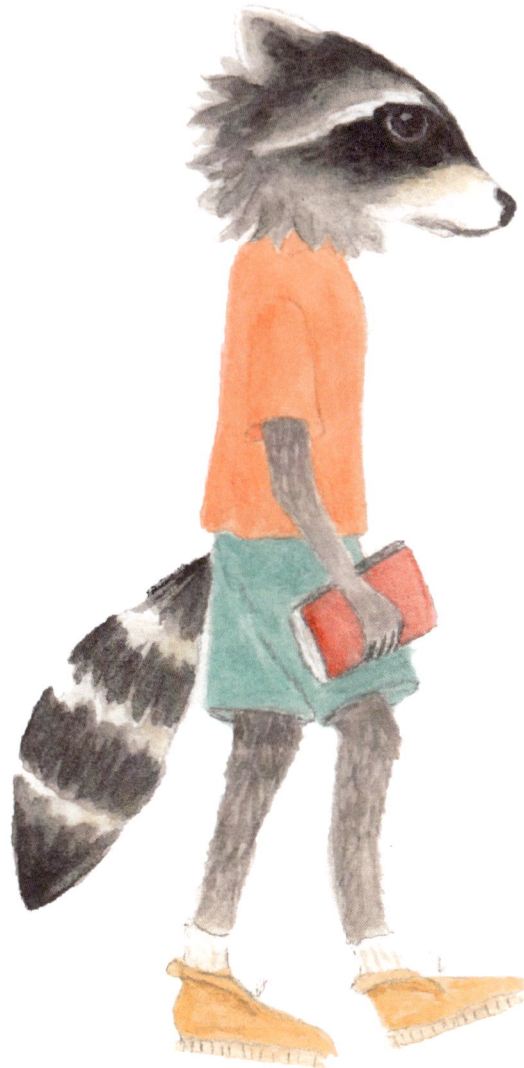

Step 2:

MINDFUL EXERCISES EXPERIENCE

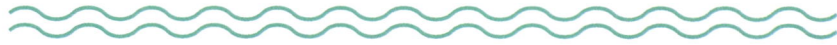

- Sit down with both feet on the ground
- Mindful Breathing:
  Inhale to the count of four.
  Exhale to the Count of five.
  Repeat four times.

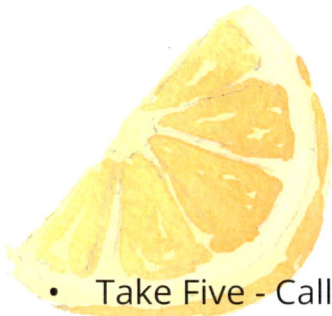

- Take Five - Call out:
  1. FIVE things that you can see
  2. FOUR things that you can touch
  3. THREE things that you can hear
  4. TWO things that you can smell
  5. ONE SOUR or TART thing that you can taste

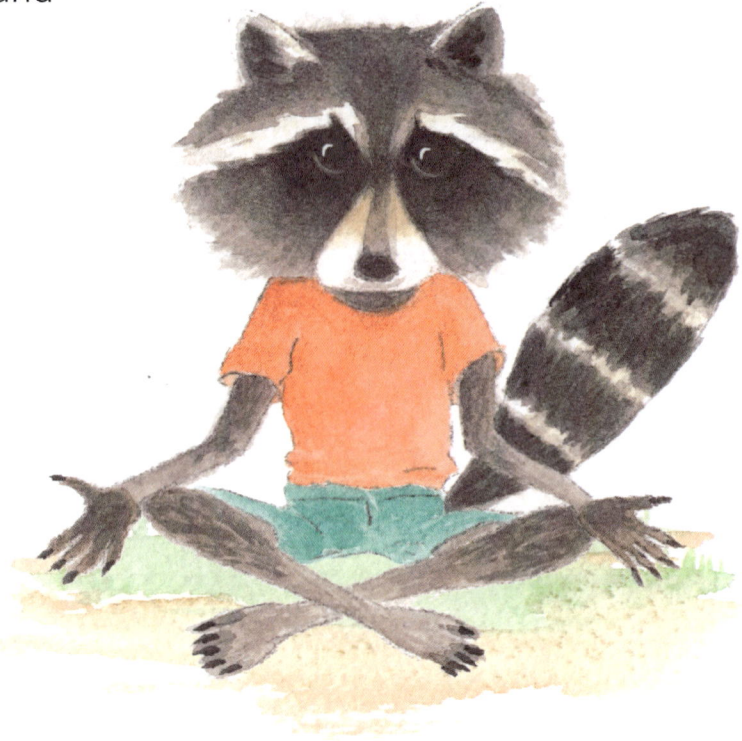

- Repeat Mindful Breathing:
  Inhale to the count of four.
  Exhale to the Count of five.
  Repeat four times.

ASK Yourself: *Am I feeling Centered and CALM?*

NO? REPEAT STEP TWO

YES? Go to STEP THREE

Step 3:

ACTION PLAN AND WHAT I LEARNED

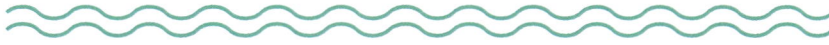

~~~~~~~~~~~~~~~~~~~~~~~~~~~~~~~~~~~~~~

- Go back to STEP ONE in your Journal and address the TRIGGER.

- How do I solve this problem? How do I prevent this from happening again?

> **Write down your insights and solutions in your Journal.**

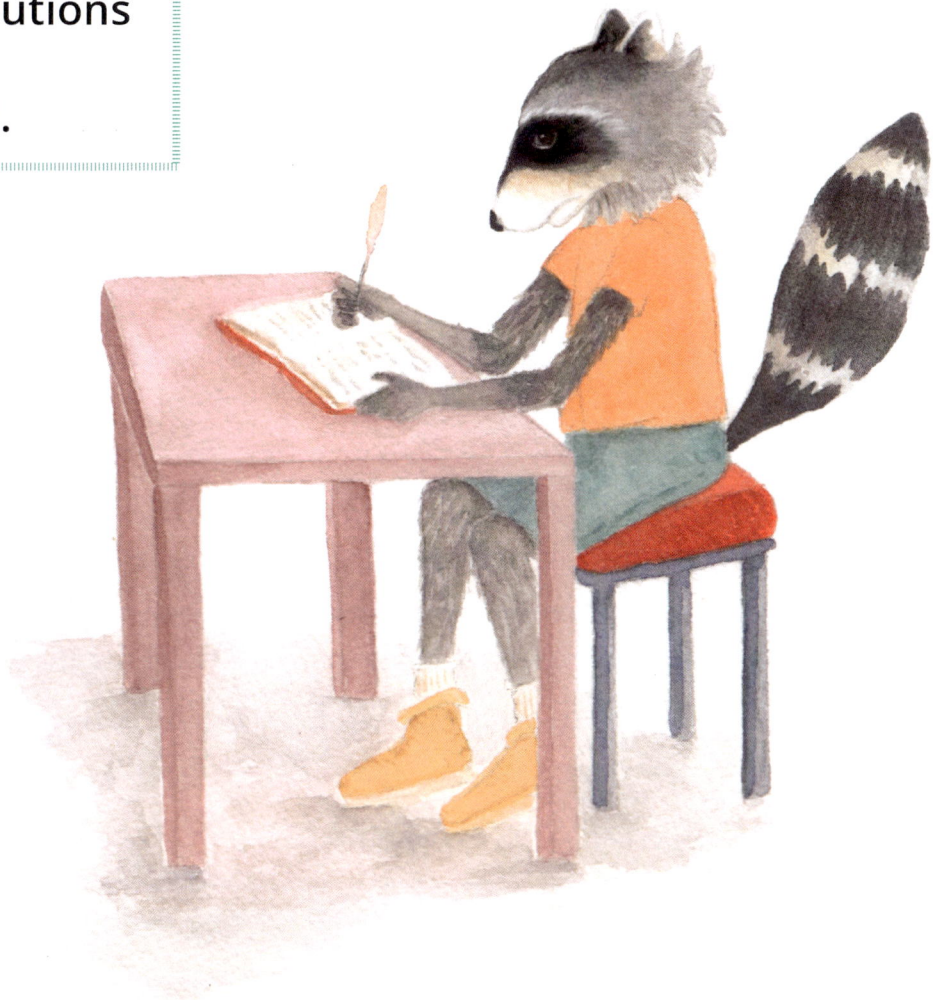

EMBRACE THE WAVE

Journaling Log

Date:

Time:

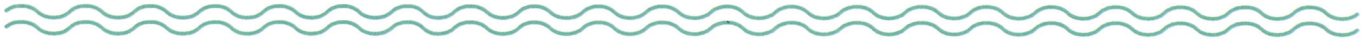

Step 1: (a) I'm feeling these emotions? (b) What was the Trigger?

_____

_____

Step 2: Mindful Exercise Experience?

_____

_____

Step 3: (a) Address the Trigger (b) My Action Plan Is? (c) What did I learn?

_____

_____

_____

_____

_____

_____

_____

EMBRACE THE WAVE

Journaling Log

Date:

Time:

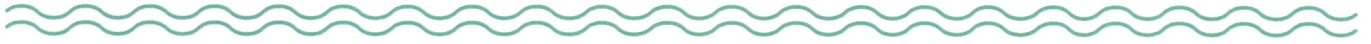

Step 1: (a) I'm feeling these emotions? (b) What was the Trigger?

_____

_____

Step 2: Mindful Exercise Experience?

_____

_____

Step 3: (a) Address the Trigger (b) My Action Plan Is? (c) What did I learn?

_____

_____

_____

_____

_____

_____

_____

EMBRACE THE WAVE

Journaling Log

Date:

Time:

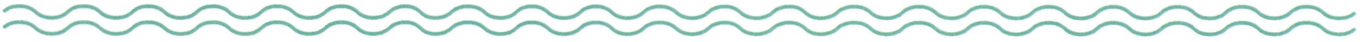

Step 1: (a) I'm feeling these emotions? (b) What was the Trigger?

_____

_____

Step 2: Mindful Exercise Experience?

_____

_____

Step 3: (a) Address the Trigger (b) My Action Plan Is? (c) What did I learn?

_____

_____

_____

_____

_____

_____

_____

EMBRACE THE WAVE

Journaling Log

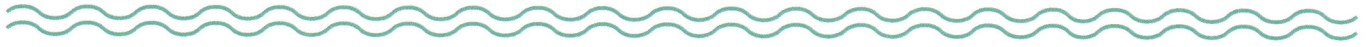

Step 1: (a) I'm feeling these emotions? (b) What was the Trigger?

_____

_____

Step 2: Mindful Exercise Experience?

_____

_____

Step 3: (a) Address the Trigger (b) My Action Plan Is? (c) What did I learn?

_____

_____

_____

_____

_____

_____

_____

EMBRACE THE WAVE

Journaling Log

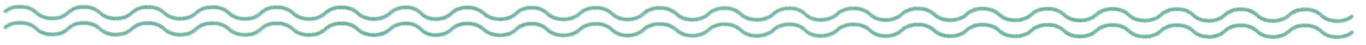

Step 1: (a) I'm feeling these emotions? (b) What was the Trigger?

_____

_____

Step 2: Mindful Exercise Experience?

_____

_____

Step 3: (a) Address the Trigger (b) My Action Plan Is? (c) What did I learn?

_____

_____

_____

_____

_____

_____

_____

EMBRACE THE WAVE

Journaling Log

Date:

Time:

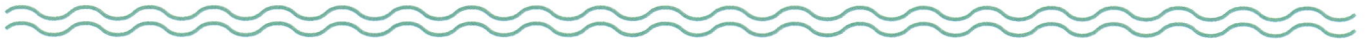

Step 1: (a) I'm feeling these emotions? (b) What was the Trigger?

_____

_____

Step 2: Mindful Exercise Experience?

_____

_____

Step 3: (a) Address the Trigger (b) My Action Plan Is? (c) What did I learn?

_____

_____

_____

_____

_____

_____

_____

Journaling Log

Date:

Time:

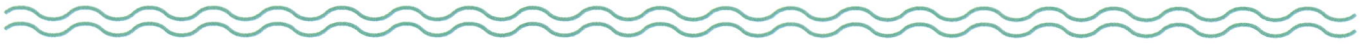

Step 1: (a) I'm feeling these emotions? (b) What was the Trigger?

_____

_____

Step 2: Mindful Exercise Experience?

_____

_____

Step 3: (a) Address the Trigger (b) My Action Plan Is? (c) What did I learn?

_____

_____

_____

_____

_____

_____

_____

EMBRACE THE WAVE

Journaling Log

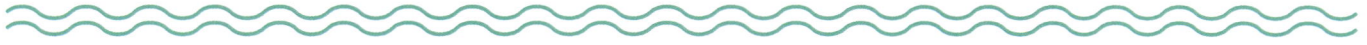

Step 1: (a) I'm feeling these emotions? (b) What was the Trigger?

_____

_____

Step 2: Mindful Exercise Experience?

_____

_____

Step 3: (a) Address the Trigger (b) My Action Plan Is? (c) What did I learn?

_____

_____

_____

_____

_____

_____

_____

EMBRACE THE WAVE

Journaling Log

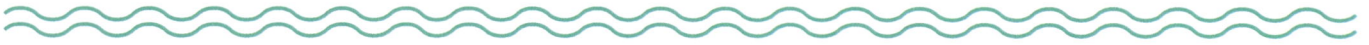

Step 1: (a) I'm feeling these emotions? (b) What was the Trigger?

_____

_____

Step 2: Mindful Exercise Experience?

_____

_____

Step 3: (a) Address the Trigger (b) My Action Plan Is? (c) What did I learn?

_____

_____

_____

_____

_____

_____

_____

EMBRACE THE WAVE

Journaling Log

Date:

Time:

~~~~~~~~~~~~~~~~~~~~~~~~~~~~~~~~~~~~~

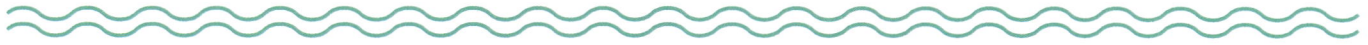

Step 1: (a) I'm feeling these emotions? (b) What was the Trigger?

_____

_____

Step 2: Mindful Exercise Experience?

_____

_____

Step 3: (a) Address the Trigger (b) My Action Plan Is? (c) What did I learn?

_____

_____

_____

_____

_____

_____

_____

Dedication

This book is dedicated to my fabulous friends and family who have supported my vision to "Develop family and child friendly resource materials to help manage and treat anxiety and distressed emotions."

www.ingramcontent.com/pod-product-compliance
Lightning Source LLC
Chambersburg PA
CBRC091037050426
42335CB00048B/207